INFLUENZA AND FLU CHALLENGES: BEYOND THE SNEEZES

Navigating the Terrain of Influenza and Unraveling the Complexities and Strategies for Resilience

BY

Daniel D. Belser

TABLE OF CONTENTS

INTRODUCTION

Welcome to "Influenza and Flu Challenges: Beyond the Sneezes." Few adversaries in the field of infectious illnesses have persistently demanded our attention and vigilance as influenza has. Sickness is often associated with sniffles and sneezing, but there is much more to it than that. There are complex biological relationships, worldwide effects, and social issues to consider. This book is an investigation into the core of influenza, with the goal of revealing its complex nature, examining its historical background, and illuminating the frequently disregarded facets of the illness that go beyond its early symptoms.

Examining the basic elements of influenza in the first chapter establishes the framework. Beyond the surface level, readers will get a thorough grasp of this seemingly familiar enemy, including the structure of the virus, its different strains, and the mechanisms that drive its transmission. In the chapters that follow, we take a historical tour through notable influenza epidemics that have had a lasting impact on cultures across time. Through examining the historical trajectory of influenza, we aim to derive significant knowledge and understanding that can guide our response to present and upcoming obstacles.

The Scope and Objectives of Our Journey

This book offers a guided exploration of the complex web of influenza and its difficulties, not just a list of facts. In addition to stressing the significance of comprehending the virus as a whole and addressing the wider ramifications that transcend beyond the immediate symptoms, the third chapter explains the scope and goals of our trip.

As we set out on this investigation, we intend to provide readers with a more informed understanding of influenza. Beyond the sniffles, we cordially welcome you to work with us to dissect the intricacies, battle unseen obstacles, and investigate groundbreaking remedies that open the door to a future immune to influenza and better equipped to fend for itself.

CHAPTER ONE

The Biology of Influenza

The biology of influenza tells a fascinating tale of a highly contagious and adaptive virus. Fundamentally, influenza is divided into three types: A, B, and C. These subtypes are identified by distinct genetic traits. This basic investigation lays the groundwork for a deeper comprehension of the global impact, difficulties, and potential therapies that go beyond the obvious symptoms and sneezes connected to this persistently difficult viral infection as we uncover the biology of influenza.

1.1 Influenza Virus Types and Subtypes

Influenza A:

Influenza A viruses are the most adaptable and often seen form. They can infect humans and a wide range of animals, such as pigs and birds. Hemagglutinin (H) and neuraminidase (N), two surface proteins that result in several subtypes, highlight their genetic diversity.

Variants of Influenza A:

The H and N protein combinations of influenza A viruses are used to further classify them. Seasonal flu outbreaks in humans, for example, have been linked to the H1N1 and H3N2 subtypes. Different influenza viruses infect a single host and exchange genetic material through a process known as genetic reassortment, which gives rise to the variety in these subtypes.

Influenza B:

Compared to influenza A, influenza B viruses primarily infect humans and have a more stable genome. They do not have as many subtypes as influenza A, despite the fact that they can still generate seasonal outbreaks.

Influenza C: Influenza C viruses can infect both humans and pigs, but they are less prevalent and usually cause a milder respiratory infection. Their surface features a unique glycoprotein that makes them identifiable.
Influenza D:

Although Influenza A, B, and C are frequently the most well-known, Influenza D is a lesser-known influenza relative that has mostly been found in cattle. Its natural host usually has moderate respiratory symptoms, but its propensity for genetic reassortment raises concerns about its potential future effects on animal and human health.

It is essential for pandemic preparedness, vaccine research, and surveillance to comprehend influenza virus types and subtypes. By deciphering the genomic complexities of these viruses, researchers can more accurately predict the possibility of antigenic drift and shift, guaranteeing that vaccination programs and public health initiatives continue to be flexible in response to influenza's always-changing landscape.

1.2 Key differences between Influenza A and Influenza B:

Host Range:

Influenza A may infect a wide variety of animals, including humans, birds, and some mammals like pigs.
Influenza B: Unlike Influenza A, it mostly affects humans and has a smaller host range.

Genetic Diversity:

Influenza A demonstrates a notable degree of genetic variety and is capable of undergoing genetic reassortment, which can result in the formation of novel subtypes.
Compared to Influenza A, Influenza B typically has a less genetically diverse genome and a more stable genome.

Subtypes:

H1N1 and H3N2, for example, are further divided into subtypes according to the mix of hemagglutinin (H) and neuraminidase (N) proteins.
Influenza B: H and N protein-based subtypes do not exist. It is divided into two different lineages (B/Yamagata and B/Victoria), which have the ability to co-circulate during flu seasons.

Antigenic Drift and Shift:

Influenza A is susceptible to both antigenic shift, which results in significant alterations brought about by genetic reassortment, and antigenic drift, which is the gradual alteration of the virus. Influenza B: Has the ability to transfer antigens but not to undergo antigenic drift.

Epidemiology:

Influenza A: Because it may infect a variety of hosts, influenza A is usually the cause of more severe flu seasons and has the potential to spread to produce pandemics.
Influenza B: Typically results in milder flu seasons; although it can create epidemics, pandemics are less likely to be caused by influenza B.

Animal Reservoirs:

Influenza A is a type of virus that can be found in a variety of animal species, such as pigs and birds. It acts as a reservoir for possible genetic reassortment.
Influenza B: It mostly affects humans and does not have the animal reservoirs that Influenza A has.

1.3 Transmission and Spread

1. Airborne Transmission:

Respiratory droplets released by an infected individual when they talk, cough, or sneeze are the main way that influenza viruses spread. Congested areas have a higher risk of transmission since these droplets can spread quickly and infect those around them.

2. Surface Contamination:

Depending on the surface type, the flu virus can live there for a few hours to many days. People can come into contact with the virus by touching their face—especially the mouth, nose, or eyes—after coming into contact with contaminated surfaces.

3. Person-to-Person Contact:

Making direct physical contact, such as a hug or handshake, with an infected individual can help spread the influenza virus. Furthermore, preventing the flu is made more difficult by the fact that individuals who have it are contagious before they exhibit symptoms.

Factors Contributing to Spread:

1. Extremely Contagious Nature: Influenza viruses are extremely contagious and have the capacity to spread widely. The virus can mutate, which makes it more contagious because new strains may emerge that can resist immunity that has already developed.

2. Asymptomatic Transmission: Before showing any symptoms, an infected person can still spread the virus, which makes it difficult to quickly identify and isolate cases. An important factor in influenza's quick spread throughout populations is this asymptomatic transmission.

3. Seasonal Variability: Influenza often has a higher incidence during the winter months in temperate countries, which facilitates viral spread and survival. In tropical regions, the virus can also be active all year round.

1.4 Host Immune Response to Influenza

The influenza virus is a dangerous respiratory infection that continuously endangers human health throughout the world. In order to effectively prevent and cure influenza infections, it is imperative to comprehend the complex interactions that exist between the virus and the immune system. The host immunological response is a key component of this defense.

The innate immune response

1. Chemical and Physical Barriers: Mucus and antimicrobial peptides, as well as physical barriers like the respiratory mucosa, are the first line of defense against influenza. These defenses work to stop the virus from getting inside the body.

2. Pattern Recognition Receptors' (PRRs') Recognition:

Dendritic and macrophage cells, among other innate immune cells, express PRRs that identify certain patterns linked to the influenza virus. TLRs are important PRRs that, when they identify viral components, cause the immune system to become activated.

3. Interferon Response: Signalling proteins called interferons are released by infected cells, and they cause nearby cells to go into an antiviral state. The adaptive immune response is started by this interferon response, which also aids in stopping the virus's propagation

Adaptive Immune Response:
1. Antibody Production: The influenza virus is targeted and neutralized by antibodies produced by B cells within the adaptive immune system. These antibodies have the ability to stop viruses from entering cells and help other immune cells remove infected cells from the body.
2. T Cell-Mediated Immunity: T cells, such as helper and cytotoxic T cells, are essential for preventing influenza infections. Helper T cells support the development of antibodies and aid in the coordination of the immune response, whereas cytotoxic T cells have the ability to destroy infected cells directly.
3. Memory Immune Response: When an influenza infection is successfully treated, memory B and T cells are produced. When the same or a closely related influenza strain is reexposed, these memory cells respond quickly and precisely., contributing to immune protection.

Immune Evasion Strategies by Influenza:
1. Antigenic Variation: New influenza virus strains with distinct surface antigens evolve as a result of the regular genetic alterations that influenza viruses experience. Seasonal epidemics and sporadic pandemics can result from the virus's ability to elude preexisting immunity due to this antigenic diversity.
2. Inhibition of Immune Signalling: Influenza viruses have developed defenses against host immune signaling pathways, which restrict interferon synthesis and weaken the immune system as a whole. This aids the virus in spreading and avoiding early discovery.
The interaction between the innate and adaptive immune systems during the host immunological response to influenza is

dynamic and intricate. Although the influenza virus has developed ways to escape and sabotage these defenses, the immune system is still capable of mounting powerful defenses against the virus. study on the immune response to influenza is ongoing, and this study is essential for the development of vaccines and antiviral treatments that can boost host immunity and lessen the impact of influenza infections on the health of people worldwide.

CHAPTER TWO

2.1 Symptoms of Influenza, Flu, and Respiratory Syncytial Virus (RSV)

The respiratory system is impacted by viral illnesses such as Respiratory Syncytial Virus (RSV) and Influenza, which is also referred to as the flu. While there are some symptoms that both illnesses have in common, it is crucial to differentiate between them in order to get an accurate diagnosis and provide the right medical care. It is essential to comprehend the symptoms linked to every virus in order to diagnose it early and take appropriate action.

Flu and Influenza Symptoms:

1. Fever: The abrupt onset of a high temperature is one of the primary signs and symptoms of influenza and flu. Chills and body aches are common symptoms of fever, which add to the general feeling of being unwell.
2. Cough: One of the most typical respiratory symptoms of influenza is a chronic cough. As the infection worsens, the cough frequently gets worse. Sometimes it becomes dry or produces phlegm.
3. Sore Throat: As a result of irritation and inflammation in the throat, influenza viruses can induce a sore throat. Swallowing difficulties frequently coexist with this symptom.

4. Fatigue: Serious exhaustion and weakness are common symptoms of influenza. This exhaustion may last for a few weeks after other symptoms have gone away.

5. Headache: During influenza infections, people frequently complain of severe headaches. The headache may be mild, moderate, or severe, and sinus congestion may be present.

6. Muscle and Joint Pain: Common influenza symptoms include aches and pains in the muscles and joints. These sores, which are frequently characterized as deep, can greatly increase the amount of discomfort felt throughout the disease.

7. Nasal congestion: Runny or stuffy noses are a common side effect of influenza viruses. Sneezing and sinus pressure may accompany this symptom.

.

Symptoms of Respiratory Syncytial Virus (RSV):

1. Sneezing and Coughing: RSV mostly affects the respiratory system, which results in symptoms like sneezing and coughing. In certain instances, wheezing may accompany the cough.

2. Runny Nose: RSV can induce nasal congestion and a runny nose, much like influenza. This is a common symptom, especially in young children and newborns.

3. Fever: Though the intensity might vary, fever is a common sign of RSV. It is possible for infants and elderly people to have higher temperatures.

4. Breathing Problems: RSV can cause serious breathing problems in certain situations, particularly in newborns and young children. Breathing quickly or difficulty could be a sign of this.

5. Decreased Appetite: Babies and early kids with RSV may have a decreased appetite, which will result in less food and drink consumption.

6. Irritability: RSV infections, particularly in young children, can result in irritability. This could be the result of respiratory issues causing discomfort.

It is crucial to identify the signs of influenza, the flu, and RSV in order to receive prompt medical attention and diagnosis. Despite the similarities between various respiratory illnesses, each one also has distinctive qualities that can aid medical experts in differentiating between them. Early diagnosis and treatment of these viral infections can improve prognoses and lower the risk of consequences, especially in susceptible groups like elderly people and newborns. Getting medical help is essential for a comprehensive examination and treatment if someone has severe or ongoing symptoms.

2.2 Overview of Antiviral Medications

1. Oseltamivir (Tamiflu): One of the antiviral drugs for influenza that is most frequently prescribed is oseltamivir. It is a member of the neuraminidase inhibitor medication class, which targets the neuraminidase enzyme found on the surface of influenza viruses. Oseltamivir slows the propagation of the virus in the body by blocking neuraminidase, which stops infected cells from releasing new viral particles.

2. Zanamivir (Relenza): Given by inhalation, Zanamivir is another neuraminidase inhibitor. Similar to oseltamivir, it stops

neuraminidase from doing its job, which stops new influenza virus particles from being released. Zanamivir is frequently recommended for people who might have trouble swallowing pills.

3. "Rapivab", also known as peramivir
The intravenous neuraminidase inhibitor peramivir has been licensed for the treatment of acute, uncomplicated influenza in people two years of age and older. For those who are unable to take oral or inhalation medicine, it is given in a medical setting and offers an option.

Mechanisms of Action: In order to prevent the virus from replicating and spreading throughout the body, antiviral drugs for influenza generally target particular viral enzymes. Neuraminidase inhibitors specifically block the neuraminidase enzyme on the surface of influenza viruses. Examples of these inhibitors are zanamivir, peramivir, and oseltamivir. The discharge of freshly produced viral particles from infected cells depends on this enzyme.

Timing of Antiviral Treatment:
Early in the course of an influenza illness, antiviral drug effectiveness is particularly significant. Although benefits may still be shown when treatment is started later in some circumstances, treatment should ideally start within 48 hours of the commencement of symptoms. Antiviral therapy is especially crucial for people who are more vulnerable to problems, such as small children, the elderly, pregnant women, and people with underlying medical issues.

Preventive Use and Prophylaxis:

In certain circumstances, antiviral drugs can also be used prophylactically to prevent influenza. When there is an influenza outbreak in an institutional setting or for people who are in close contact with confirmed patients, this strategy is frequently taken into account.

Antiviral drugs are essential for treating influenza and the flu because they lessen the illness's symptoms, lessen its effects, and avoid complications. Oseltamivir, zanamivir, and peramivir are examples of neuraminidase inhibitors, which are the cornerstone of antiviral therapy. Medical specialists evaluate each patient's situation to determine the best course of action, including when to take medication. For the greatest outcomes, people who are more likely to experience problems should seek medical help as soon as possible and follow the suggested treatment plan when taking antiviral drugs.

2.3 Challenges in Antiviral Treatment

Although antiviral drugs have demonstrated efficacy in reducing the symptoms of influenza and the flu, there are still a number of difficulties in treating them. In order to maximize the use of antiviral medications, improve treatment results, and lower the incidence of influenza-related sickness and consequences, these issues must be resolved.

1. Antiviral Resistance: The emergence of antiviral resistance poses a serious obstacle to the treatment of influenza. Antiviral drugs may become less effective as a result of influenza virus mutations over time. Resistance to neuraminidase inhibitors, including zanamivir and oseltamivir, has been observed; this

highlights the necessity of continued monitoring and the creation of novel antiviral medications.

2. Treatment Timing: Antiviral drugs work best when used early in the course of an influenza infection, preferably within 48 hours after the onset of symptoms. However, the prompt beginning of antiviral treatment can be hampered, decreasing its effectiveness, by delayed diagnosis or delayed presentation to medical facilities.

3. Limited Treatment choices: The necessity for expanding treatment choices for influenza is underscored by the limited number of antiviral drugs that have been approved and resistance issues. Increasing the number of antiviral medications with distinct modes of action can offer substitutes for people who might not react well to current treatments.

4. Vaccination Gaps: One factor contributing to the difficulties with antiviral therapy is the incomplete vaccination rate for influenza. Vaccination is still the best protective measure. People who are not vaccinated or who have not had sufficient vaccination may be more susceptible to serious sickness and require antiviral medication.

5. High-Risk Populations: Treating and identifying high-risk groups is essential to avoiding serious problems. These groups include small children, the elderly, pregnant women, and people with underlying medical disorders. It is difficult to provide these susceptible populations with prompt access to antiviral drugs.

6. Public Awareness and Healthcare-Seeking Behavior: therapy start may be delayed during influenza epidemics due to a lack of public knowledge of the significance of early antiviral therapy and healthcare-seeking behavior. In order to encourage quick

medical attention for suspected influenza illnesses, improved public education campaigns are required.

7. Global Surveillance and Preparedness: Because influenza viruses can vary widely around the world, surveillance is crucial for tracking circulating strains and identifying new dangers. Obstacles in worldwide monitoring and readiness could delay the prompt creation of antiviral drugs specific to novel and developing influenza viruses.

8. Cost and Accessibility: The pricing and accessibility of antiviral drugs may provide challenges, especially in resource-poor areas. Assuring the availability and equitable distribution of antiviral drugs is crucial for global influenza control programs.

2.4 Does the flu shot protect against influenza?

Indeed, the purpose of the flu vaccination is to prevent influenza. Every year, a vaccination known as the flu shot is created to defend against particular strains of the influenza virus that are predicted to be common during flu season. The vaccination elicits an immunological response from the body that includes the creation of antibodies that are capable of identifying and combating influenza viruses.

It's crucial to remember that the influenza virus can change and that various strains may be prevalent during each flu season, making the vaccination ineffective in 100% of cases. Still, the vaccine can lessen the intensity of the disease, avoid complications, and cut the risk of hospitalization and death even in the case that a person who has gotten the shot gets the flu later on.

It is advised to have a flu shot every year, particularly for those who are in high-risk categories like small children, the elderly, pregnant women, and people with underlying medical disorders. The vaccination decreases the general spread of the flu among the population by promoting communal immunity in addition to individual protection.

Emerging Therapeutic Approaches

Research and development efforts are focused on developing novel therapeutic approaches for influenza and flu, with the goal of tackling issues such as treatment options being restricted and antiviral resistance. A potentially fruitful path is the investigation of host-targeted treatments, which instead of going after the virus directly target the host's biological response to viral infections. This strategy aims to improve the immune system's capacity to fight influenza, which may lower the likelihood of developing antiviral resistance. Furthermore, because they specifically target components of the influenza virus, developments in the field of monoclonal antibodies hold promise for both therapy and prevention. To increase medication efficacy and decrease side effects, solutions based on nanotechnology are being researched. Examples of these tactics include drug delivery systems and nanoparticle antivirals. These new therapeutic strategies provide hope for more varied and potent treatment options as research advances, which will ultimately help create a more resilient and flexible response to influenza and flu outbreaks.

CHAPTER THREE

3.1 Long-Term Effects of Influenza and Flu

The possibility that influenza may have long-term consequences on people that extend beyond the acute stage of the illness is becoming more widely acknowledged. Comprehensive patient care, public health planning, and additional study into the long-term effects of influenza infections all depend on an understanding of these lasting effects.

1. Post-Infectious Complications: After recovering from the flu, some people may have post-infectious complications. These can include secondary bacterial infections that cause sinusitis, pneumonia, or ear infections. These can make healing take longer and lead to chronic health problems.

2. Respiratory Effects: People with severe influenza infections are more often recognized to have long-term respiratory complications. The flu may worsen or provoke long-term symptoms and reduce lung function in people with chronic respiratory diseases including asthma or chronic obstructive pulmonary disease (COPD).

3. Cardiovascular Complications: Research points to a possible connection between serious influenza infections and

cardiovascular issues. People who have had the flu in the past, especially those who already have cardiovascular issues, may be more vulnerable to heart attacks, strokes, or other cardiovascular events in the months that follow the infection.

4. Neurological and Cognitive Effects: A new study suggests that influenza may have negative effects on the nervous system and the brain. After severe flu infections, some people suffer persistent cognitive impairments, memory issues, or mood swings; however, the processes causing these consequences are still being studied.

5. Fatigue and Malaise: People recuperating from influenza frequently report experiencing prolonged fatigue and a generalized feeling of malaise as long-term side effects. This chronic fatigue, which can occasionally last for weeks or even months following the acute stage of the illness, can have an adverse effect on everyday functioning and quality of life.

6. Effect on Mental Health: Influenza can have a physical and mental health toll. Stress from the disease and its aftermath may contribute to elevated levels of anxiety, sadness, or other mental health issues in some people both during and after they recover from the flu.

7. Immunological Consequences: Severe influenza infections may modify the body's capacity to fight off subsequent infections by permanently affecting the immune system. Determining long-term immunity and providing guidance for vaccine development requires an understanding of these immunological effects.

8. Risk of Complications in Vulnerable Populations: Depending on how severe their influenza infections are, a number of

groups, including the elderly, small children, pregnant women, and those with underlying medical issues, may be more vulnerable to long-term complications. Comprehensive healthcare must recognize and meet the unique requirements of these vulnerable populations.

Despite the common belief that influenza is a transient illness, there is growing evidence that influenza may have long-term consequences that go beyond the acute stage. In order to give patients recuperating from influenza the proper care and support, healthcare professionals must be aware of these effects. To reduce the flu's negative impacts on general health and well-being, more study on the long-term effects of influenza is necessary. The implementation of public health campaigns and preventative measures, such as vaccination programs, is crucial in mitigating the severity of influenza illnesses and limiting their long-term consequences.

3.2 How long does influenza last in Children and Adults?

A person's age, general health, and the particular strain of the influenza virus that is causing the illness can all have an impact on how long influenza, sometimes known as the flu, lasts. Little children, elderly people, and those with compromised immune systems typically experience more severe and extended flu symptoms.

1. Children: Flu symptoms usually last in children for a few days to roughly a week. For a longer amount of time, some kids, nevertheless, can continue to feel weak, exhausted, or have a persistent cough. Pneumonia or subsequent bacterial infections are examples of consequences that might worsen a bout of disease. It's imperative that parents and other carers keep an eye

on their child's symptoms, make sure they stay hydrated and seek medical assistance if the child's breathing becomes difficult or if symptoms increase.

2. Adults: Within a week, healthy adults typically experience a reduction in flu-related symptoms. On the other hand, symptoms like weakness, exhaustion, and a persistent cough could last for another week or two. Adults may occasionally suffer from post-viral fatigue, which is characterized by persistent weakness and exhaustion after the initial sickness has subsided. The length of the sickness can be prolonged by complications, and older persons or those with underlying medical concerns may take longer to recover.

It's crucial to remember that antiviral drugs can lessen the length and intensity of influenza symptoms if they are taken early in the disease. Those who are more likely to experience complications or a serious sickness should seek medical assistance as soon as possible because these medications work best when administered within the first 48 hours of symptom onset.

3.3 Impact on Vulnerable Populations

1. Elderly Population: Serious influenza-related complications are more likely to occur in the elderly, particularly those 65 and older. The immune system's ability to mount a successful defense may be compromised by immunosenescence or age-related decreases in immunological function. In addition to an increased risk of hospitalization and mortality from flu-related complications, this population is more vulnerable to pneumonia and the worsening of pre-existing chronic illnesses.

2. Little ones: Young children are more susceptible to the flu, particularly those under the age of five. Due to their immature immune systems and limited history of flu strain exposure, they are more vulnerable to serious illnesses, respiratory distress, and follow-up conditions such as pneumonia and ear infections. A higher hospitalization rate in young children can also be caused by influenza.

3. Pregnant Women: Immune and respiratory system modifications during pregnancy increase a woman's vulnerability to serious influenza infections. Preterm birth, low birth weight, and complications like pneumonia are among the threats that the flu can offer to both the growing fetus and the pregnant woman.

4. People with Chronic Health illnesses: People who have underlying medical illnesses, such as diabetes, cardiovascular disease, immunosuppressive disorders, or chronic respiratory diseases (such as asthma or COPD), are more susceptible to serious influenza-related consequences. The flu can worsen pre-existing diseases, increasing the risk of hospitalization, extended recovery times, and even death.

5. Immunocompromised Individuals: People who have compromised immune systems, either from illnesses or immunosuppressive therapies (such as organ transplants or chemotherapy), are at a higher risk of developing severe influenza complications. Longer sickness duration and a higher risk of complications can arise from a weakened immune response.

6. Socioeconomically Disadvantaged Groups: In addition to impediments to immunization, congested living circumstances, and restricted access to healthcare are some of the other challenges that vulnerable communities may encounter. All of

these things raise the chance of getting sick from influenza, increase the danger of exposure, and delay getting medical attention.

7. Effect on Mental Health: For susceptible groups, the effects of influenza go beyond physical health. The possibility of a severe illness, complications, and long-term repercussions from influenza can cause stress and anxiety, which can exacerbate mental health issues in these populations.

The impact that influenza has on vulnerable communities highlights the significance of focused public health initiatives, immunization programs, and easily available healthcare. Protecting the health and well-being of these at-risk populations requires targeted measures including vaccination campaigns and early medical intervention that aim to lower the risk of influenza. In order to lessen the effects of influenza and improve health outcomes for these populations, a comprehensive strategy that takes into account the special requirements and difficulties faced by vulnerable groups is necessary.

3.4 Co-Infections and Complications

Although the flu can cause a number of difficulties on its own, co-infections with other viruses can make the sickness much worse. Healthcare providers must be aware of the possibility of co-infections and the symptoms of influenza in order to give thorough care and reduce unfavorable outcomes.
1. Bacterial Co-Infections: Especially in the respiratory system, influenza can foster an environment that is favorable for bacterial co-infections. Common consequences of influenza include secondary bacterial infections, which can lead to

pneumonia, sinusitis, or ear infections. Haemophilus influenza, Staphylococcus aureus, and Streptococcus pneumonia are a few of the bacteria that are commonly linked to these co-infections.

2. Viral Co-Infections:

Simultaneous co-infections with other respiratory viruses, such as adenovirus, rhinovirus, or respiratory syncytial virus (RSV), can worsen respiratory symptoms and lengthen sickness. Multiple virus infections might make identification and treatment more difficult.

3. Exacerbation of Chronic Disorders: Asthma, diabetes, cardiovascular disease, and chronic obstructive pulmonary disease (COPD) are just a few of the chronic health disorders that influenza can aggravate. Patients who have these underlying diseases may see a longer recovery time, a worsening of symptoms, and an increased chance of hospitalization.

4. Myocarditis and Pericarditis: Severe influenza outbreaks may result in inflammation of the heart (myocarditis) or the pericardium (pericarditis). Breathlessness, chest pain, and, in severe situations, heart failure can be caused by these issues. People who already have heart problems are especially susceptible to these consequences.

5. Respiratory Distress Syndrome: Acute respiratory distress syndrome (ARDS), a potentially fatal illness marked by a sudden onset of severe respiratory failure, can develop from influenza in extreme circumstances. Mechanical breathing and intensive care support may be necessary for ARDS patients.

6. Neurological Complications: Although they are uncommon, meningitis or encephalitis are two neurological conditions that influenza can cause. These illnesses can cause symptoms

including disorientation, seizures, or excruciating headaches, which call for quick medical intervention.

7. Secondary Bacterial Pneumonia: The influenza virus weakens the respiratory epithelium, increasing a person's susceptibility to bacterial invasion. This is why influenza-associated pneumonia is a serious consequence. Morbidity and mortality rates can rise sharply as a result of secondary bacterial pneumonia.

8. Dehydration and Electrolyte Imbalance: Fever, sweating, and decreased fluid intake are common flu symptoms. Dehydration and electrolyte imbalances can develop in severe cases, which can result in problems such as kidney dysfunction and, in the worst situations, multi-organ failure.

9. Enhanced Risk in Vulnerable Populations: People with underlying medical disorders, the elderly, small children, pregnant women, and people with compromised immune systems are among the vulnerable groups that are more susceptible to the complications of influenza and co-infections. Effective management requires recognizing and meeting these groups' particular demands.

Co-infections and influenza-related complications draw attention to the disease's complexity and stress the value of early detection, preventive measures, and prompt treatment. The major method of lowering the risk of influenza and its complications is still vaccination. In order to guarantee the best possible outcomes for patients and reduce the burden of influenza-related disease, healthcare professionals are essential in identifying and managing co-infections and consequences, especially in more susceptible populations.

CHAPTER FOUR

4.1 Surveillance and Early Detection

In order to effectively monitor and contain epidemics, surveillance, and early detection are essential elements of influenza and flu management. Quick detection of influenza cases and tracking of virus strains in circulation allow public health officials, medical experts, and legislators to take appropriate action, stop the spread of the illness, and safeguard susceptible groups. This all-encompassing surveillance approach uses a variety of techniques and instruments to identify and monitor influenza activity on a local, national, and international scale.

1. Clinical Surveillance: Clinical surveillance is keeping an eye out for cases of severe acute respiratory infections (SARI) or influenza-like illness (ILI) in healthcare settings. The number of cases reported by healthcare providers is analyzed to determine geographic patterns, trends, and the intensity of influenza activity. Reports in a timely manner facilitate resource allocation, intervention planning, and public health action implementation by authorities.

2. Laboratory Surveillance: This method is essential for verifying influenza cases, figuring out viral strains, and spotting any antigenic alterations in the viruses that are in circulation. Rapid antigen testing and polymerase chain reaction (PCR) are

two diagnostic techniques that are used to identify influenza viruses in respiratory specimens. Monitoring laboratory-confirmed cases yields useful information for selecting vaccine strains and tracking antiviral resistance.

3. Virological Surveillance: To identify the prevalent strains of influenza virus circulating in a particular season, influenza virus specimens are collected and analyzed as part of virological surveillance. To guarantee that annual influenza vaccinations offer the best defense against circulating strains, this information is crucial for updating the shots. The sharing of virus specimens and data is made easier by international cooperation via the Global Influenza Surveillance and Response System (GISRS) of the World Health Organisation (WHO).

4. Syndromic Surveillance: Syndromic surveillance means keeping an eye on non-traditional data sources like sales of over-the-counter medications, absenteeism rates from schools, and online searches for symptoms of the flu. These markers can support conventional surveillance techniques by offering early warning signs of elevated influenza activity.

5. Pharmacological Surveillance: Sales data on antiviral drugs can reveal information about the frequency and intensity of influenza outbreaks. Public health actions and communication campaigns may be prompted by increased sales of antiviral medications, which could be a sign of increased influenza activity.

6. Molecular Epidemiology: This field of study examines the genetic makeup of influenza virus strains to learn about their evolution, patterns of transmission and possible effects on vaccination efficacy. This method aids in monitoring the arrival

and dissemination of particular strains both within and between populations.

7. International Surveillance: Since influenza is a worldwide threat, efficient surveillance and early detection necessitate international cooperation. Information, surveillance data, and virus specimens are exchanged more easily between the WHO and other international organizations in order to track influenza trends worldwide, evaluate pandemic risks, and plan vaccines.

8. Public Health Messaging and Reporting: In order to promote preventative actions, facilitate early identification, and raise public awareness, timely dissemination of surveillance data to the general public, healthcare professionals, and pertinent stakeholders is imperative. When people report with clarity and accuracy, it becomes easier for them to make educated decisions and get care as soon as they start showing signs of the flu.

Effective influenza control and prevention are based on surveillance and early detection. By combining several surveillance techniques, it is possible to get a thorough picture of influenza activity and take preventative action to lessen the effects of seasonal flu and possible pandemics. Constant advancements in data exchange, international cooperation, and monitoring technology strengthen our capacity to quickly address new influenza risks, safeguard susceptible groups, and eventually lower the worldwide incidence of influenza and flu-related diseases.

4.2 International Collaboration

Coordinated efforts and international cooperation are needed to monitor influenza outbreaks, contain them, and put effective preventative measures in place. Influenza is a worldwide health concern. Global interconnection and the cross-border transmissibility of influenza viruses highlight the significance of cooperative efforts across nations, international organizations, and research centers. This page examines the value of international cooperation in the management of influenza and related illnesses, emphasizing important elements and programs that provide a coordinated worldwide response.

1. World Health Organisation (WHO): In order to effectively coordinate global efforts to combat influenza, the World Health Organisation is essential. A global network of labs and organizations, the WHO Global Influenza Surveillance and Response System (GISRS) is in charge of keeping an eye on influenza viruses, exchanging data, and promoting research. Through this partnership, influenza epidemiology is better understood, vaccine strain selection is informed, and pandemic preparedness is supported.

2. Pandemic readiness and Response: Planning for pandemic readiness and response requires international cooperation. To make sure that nations are prepared to act swiftly and decisively in the event of the introduction of new influenza viruses with pandemic potential, the WHO collaborates with member states to create and maintain frameworks for pandemic preparedness. This covers plans for creating vaccines, dispersing antiviral medications, and communicating globally.

3. International Vaccine Distribution: Equitable influenza vaccine distribution requires international cooperation. The World Health Organisation (WHO) campaigns for greater access to vaccines, particularly in low- and middle-income countries, and encourages the sharing of vaccine-related technologies and vaccine production in various locations. Global vaccine coverage has become more effective and extensive as a result of collaborative efforts.

4. Research and Surveillance Networks: International scientists and institutions can share information and resources more easily when they work together through collaborative research networks like the Global Consortium for H5N8 and Related Influenza Viruses. By advancing our knowledge of influenza virology, epidemiology, and antiviral resistance, these networks help to create more potent preventative and therapeutic approaches.

5. Data Sharing and Open Communication: Early influenza epidemic detection and response depend heavily on data sharing and open communication between nations and international organizations. The prompt sharing of data on vaccine efficacy, circulating virus strains, and surveillance results enables nations to modify their public health policies in response to international developments.

6. capability Building and Training: The goal of collaborative projects is to increase the training and capability of laboratories and healthcare professionals across various locations. International organizations fund training initiatives that improve nations' capacities to identify, identify, and contain influenza

outbreaks, thereby fortifying global response and readiness systems.

7. Cross-Border Surveillance: Because influenza viruses transcend national boundaries, cross-border surveillance necessitates international cooperation. In order to exchange information, plan responses, and stop the spread of influenza strains among regions, neighboring nations frequently cooperate with one another. In order to manage seasonal influenza and lessen the effects of prospective pandemics, cooperation is especially crucial.

8. Public Health Campaigns: International cooperation includes public health campaigns that provide correct information to the public, encourage preventative measures, and increase public awareness. Coordinated activities guarantee messaging consistency and support the development of an international influenza preventive and control culture.

Effective management of influenza and related illnesses relies heavily on international collaboration. Countries and organizations around the world may work together to address the difficulties presented by influenza viruses by promoting partnerships, exchanging resources, and aligning strategies. In addition to strengthening the groundwork for pandemic preparedness, research improvements, and fair access to preventative measures, a coordinated worldwide response improves our capacity to identify and contain influenza epidemics. Collaboration is still essential to safeguarding public health worldwide as the influenza pandemic continues to evolve.

4.3 Public Health Measures and Communication

Effective communication and public health initiatives are essential for controlling, preventing, and lessening the effects of influenza and flu outbreaks. Public health authorities are able to promote preventative measures, educate the public, and act quickly in the event of a developing concern by putting focused policies into action and keeping open lines of communication. This page examines the most important public health precautions and communication tactics used in managing influenza and the flu, emphasizing their importance in maintaining public health.

1. Vaccination Campaigns: Public health authorities around the world hold yearly vaccination campaigns since immunization is the cornerstone of influenza prevention. The public is primarily educated on the value of vaccinations, myths are debunked, and concerns are addressed through communication campaigns. Transparent and easily obtainable information promotes mass vaccination, safeguarding people and bolstering immunity within the community.

2. Public Awareness Campaigns: To inform the public about influenza symptoms, transmission routes, and preventative measures, public health organizations showcase awareness campaigns. To reach a variety of consumers, these campaigns make use of a range of media platforms, such as printed materials, radio, television, and social media. The messaging stresses the value of staying at home when unwell, maintaining good hand hygiene, and respiratory etiquette.

3. Hygiene and Respiratory Etiquette: In order to stop the transmission of influenza viruses, it is crucial to encourage basic hygiene behaviors including frequent hand washing and covering sneezes and coughs. The emphasis of public health communication is on these steps to lower the risk of transmission in homes, workplaces, and public areas.

4. Early Detection and Testing Guidance: People are more likely to seek prompt medical assistance when they are aware of the significance of early detection and testing for influenza symptoms. Public health announcements urge people with flu-like symptoms to get in touch with medical professionals as soon as possible. This allows for an early diagnosis and suitable treatment.

5. Antiviral Medication Awareness: Public health messaging emphasizes the use of antiviral drugs in treating influenza, particularly in high-risk patients. The significance of early treatment is emphasized for those who are more vulnerable to complications, including the elderly, small children, and people with existing medical disorders.

6. School and Workplace Guidance: Public health officials advise schools and workplaces on how to stop the spread of influenza. To stop the virus from spreading in enclosed spaces, this includes guidelines for immunization, the implementation of respiratory hygiene precautions, and absenteeism management strategies.

7. Travel warnings: Public health organizations release travel warnings and guidelines to lower the risk of influenza

transmission across international boundaries during flu seasons and pandemics. In order to protect themselves and others, travelers are provided with information on preventive measures, including vaccinations and good hygiene habits.

8. Emergency Preparedness and Response Communication: During public health emergencies, such as influenza pandemics, effective communication is essential. Information on the changing situation, treatment choices, preventive measures, and other public health interventions are promptly disseminated by authorities. Effective and clear communication promotes adherence to suggested actions and helps establish trust.

9. Crisis Communication Plans: During influenza epidemics, public health organizations create and carry out crisis communication plans to respond to public concerns and provide factual information. These plans include debunking myths, addressing uncertainties, and developing communication tactics for various stages of an outbreak.

10. Community Engagement and Partnerships: Public health messages are more effective when they are developed in conjunction with local organizations, healthcare practitioners, and community leaders. Cooperation ensures that messages are addressed to a variety of audiences, take into account cultural differences, and meet particular needs in the community.

In order to manage influenza and the flu, public health initiatives and communication are essential because they support early detection, coordinated interventions, and prevention. Public health authorities enable people to take proactive measures to safeguard themselves and their communities by providing clear and accessible communication. Public health initiatives support a robust and knowledgeable worldwide response to influenza outbreaks by encouraging cooperation, openness, and community involvement.

CHAPTER FIVE

5.1 Cutting-Edge Technologies

Global researchers are always looking for novel ways to comprehend, avoid, and treat influenza. Innovative technologies are essential for furthering influenza research, offering fresh perspectives, and enabling discoveries. Here, we examine a few of the cutting-edge innovations reshaping the field of influenza research.

1. Next-Generation Sequencing (NGS):
Through the rapid and economical decoding of whole genomes, Next-Generation Sequencing has completely changed the discipline of genomics. NGS makes it possible to analyze viral genomes thoroughly for influenza research, offering insights into genetic variability, evolution, and the creation of novel strains. Scientists may track influenza viruses and anticipate possible outbreaks with the use of this technology, which supports monitoring operations.

2. Gene Editing using CRISPR-Cas9:
Targeted and accurate gene editing is now possible because of CRISPR-Cas9 technology. In order to explore certain genes and comprehend their functions in viral replication, transmission, and pathogenesis, scientists are employing CRISPR to modify the viral genome in influenza research. The creation of

innovative vaccinations and antiviral treatments appears to be promising with this technique.

3. The Computational Biology and Cryo-Electron Microscopy (Cryo-EM):
Unprecedented insights into the three-dimensional structure of influenza viruses have been made possible by developments in structural biology, notably in the field of cryo-EM. Researchers can see viral proteins and comprehend how they interact with host cells thanks to this high-resolution imaging approach. The development of medications and vaccinations that specifically target viral components requires this understanding.

4. Artificial Intelligence and Machine Learning:
Large-scale datasets produced by influenza studies are being analyzed using artificial intelligence and machine learning techniques. These technologies support the identification of patterns, the prediction of viral evolution, and the evaluation of antiviral drug efficacy. AI models are also useful in the creation of diagnostic instruments and in locating possible therapeutic targets.

5. The Technology of Virus-Like Particles (VLP):
Engineered entities that resemble the architecture of viruses but lack the genetic material of the virus are called virus-like particles. VLPs are utilized as a platform for vaccine development in influenza research. Since they don't include live or inactivated viruses, they present a less risky option than standard vaccinations in terms of adverse effects.

6. Sequencing of Single-Cell RNA:

Researchers can examine gene expression in single cells by using single-cell RNA sequencing. This technology aids in the understanding of how the virus interacts with host cells and triggers the host immune response in influenza research. A thorough grasp of single-cell dynamics can provide crucial insights into the intricate nature of the host-pathogen relationship.

7. Drug Delivery Using Nanotechnology:
The targeted delivery of antiviral medications via nanotechnology is a growing area of research. Antiviral drugs can be encapsulated in nanoparticles and delivered to targeted infected cells. This strategy possibly transforms the way influenza is treated by increasing the therapeutic benefit while reducing adverse effects.

These developments not only broaden our knowledge of the virus but also open new avenues for creative approaches to treatment, diagnosis, and prevention. The fight against influenza has become more complex as technology advances, which gives optimism for future control and mitigation tactics that will be more potent.

5.2 Breakthroughs in Understanding the Influenza Virus

Researchers have come a long way in understanding the complexity of the influenza virus throughout time. Advances in our comprehension of its molecular biology, evolution, and interactions with the host have made it possible to develop more potent preventive, therapeutic, and control measures. Here, we explore a few significant discoveries that have revolutionized our knowledge of the influenza virus.

1. Specificity of receptor binding:

One important finding in influenza research is the selectivity of the virus's receptor binding. The two essential viral proteins, hemagglutinin (HA) and neuraminidase (NA) have been found. Researchers now know how these proteins interact with host cell receptors to control the infectivity and spread of influenza viruses. This information has significant ramifications for developing vaccinations and tailored antiviral treatments.

2. Shift and Drift of Antigens:

The diversity and adaptability of influenza viruses have been largely explained by the idea of antigenic drift and shift. Antigenic drift refers to the virus's slow genetic alterations that enable it to circumvent immunity that already exists. Conversely, antigenic shift is the outcome of significant genetic reassortment, which gives rise to novel influenza strains that have the potential to cause a pandemic. It is essential to comprehend these pathways in order to anticipate and manage seasonal and pandemic influenza outbreaks.

3. Dynamics of Zoonotic Transmission:

Advances in surveillance and genetics have illuminated the dynamics of influenza virus zoonotic transmission in recent years. Scientists have discovered animal reservoirs, especially in pigs and birds, where influenza viruses can reassort genetically before spreading to human populations. Our capacity to keep an eye on and reduce the possibility of novel influenza strains arising from animal reservoirs is improved by this knowledge.

4. Variability in the Host Immune Response:

Recent developments in systems biology and immunology have revealed the finer points of the human immune response to influenza infection. Novel insights encompass comprehending the fluctuations in personal immune reactions, variables impacting vulnerability, and the evolution of immunity across temporal dimensions. The creation of more individualized and efficient vaccinations and therapies is aided by this knowledge.

5. Gaining Structural Understanding using Cryo-Electron Microscopy:

Through the use of cryo-electron microscopy, or cryo-EM, scientists have been able to see the influenza virus's three-dimensional structure at previously unheard-of resolutions. This discovery has shed light on the structures, purposes, and interactions of viral proteins with host cells. Such structural information is crucial for creating vaccinations and antiviral medications that specifically target vulnerable virus components.

6. Advances in Big Data Analysis and Surveillance:
Technological advances in surveillance and data analytics have revolutionized our capacity to track and anticipate influenza outbreaks. Large datasets containing clinical, epidemiological, and genomic data can be analyzed in real time to help with early strain detection and faster public health response.

7. Molecular-Level Interactions between Virus and Host:
Advances in research have explored the molecular details of the interactions between the influenza virus and its host. Novel targets for antiviral medication development can be found by comprehending how the virus molecularly manipulates host cell machinery and eludes immune responses.

Together, these discoveries add to our understanding of the influenza virus, making it more complex and nuanced. It is hoped that when more aspects of its biology are discovered by researchers, these discoveries may lead to improved approaches to controlling and preventing influenza, ultimately lessening the disease's worldwide burden.

5.3 Future Directions in Influenza Research

Scientists are investigating novel approaches that could lead to revolutionary discoveries in the understanding, prevention, and treatment of influenza as the field of study into the disease continues to develop. Technology breakthroughs, interdisciplinary teamwork, and a greater understanding of the intricate relationships between the virus and its hosts will influence the future paths of influenza research. Here, we summarise some of the major areas that will probably propel the next round of influenza research breakthroughs and developments.

1. Universal Influenza Vaccines:
The quest to create a vaccination against influenza that is universal is gathering steam. A universal vaccine, in contrast to the seasonal vaccinations currently in use, would offer comprehensive and durable defense against a variety of influenza strains, negating the need for yearly updates. Researchers are looking at conserved virus areas that might be targets for a universal vaccine. They are also looking into novel vaccine platforms like mRNA and viral vector-based techniques to see whether they can help accomplish this bold objective.

2. Antiviral Therapies Targeting Host Factors:

Traditional antiviral medications target specific viral components; however, future studies might concentrate on discovering and targeting host factors that are necessary for the propagation and reproduction of influenza viruses. Through the disturbance of the host-virus relationship, these treatments may offer an increased range of antiviral efficacy and a decreased risk of drug resistance.

3. Combined One Health Methods:

Influenza research is starting to place more emphasis on the interdisciplinary One Health approach, which acknowledges the interdependence of environmental, animal, and human health. Integrated surveillance systems that track influenza in both human and animal populations will probably be the focus of future research. To anticipate and stop zoonotic transmissions and possible pandemics, it is essential to comprehend the dynamics of influenza in many species.

4. Harnessing Artificial Intelligence for Prediction and Surveillance:

The field of influenza research is expected to benefit greatly from developments in machine learning and artificial intelligence (AI). These tools can improve real-time surveillance, detect new strains of the virus, forecast influenza patterns, and analyze enormous datasets. Antiviral medications and vaccines may be designed with greater efficacy thanks to AI models, which can anticipate prospective therapeutic targets and optimize vaccination formulations.

5. Personalised and Customised Vaccines:

Future studies on influenza could look towards creating individualized, customized vaccinations for particular people or demographics. To maximize the effectiveness of vaccines, this strategy might take into account variables including age, immunological condition, and genetic differences. Vaccines that are tailored to an individual's health have the potential to increase vaccination coverage and help better contain influenza outbreaks.

6. Cutting-Edge Medication Delivery Systems:

Nanotechnology and tailored delivery techniques are two examples of innovations in medication delivery systems that may increase the efficacy of antiviral treatments while reducing side effects. These developments could result in more effective medication delivery to infected cells, enhancing the prognosis for influenza patients.

7. Recognising Immunity and Long-Term Effects:

There is a growing body of research on the durability of immunity and the long-term repercussions of influenza infection. Public health policies and vaccination programs will be more informed if they take into account how the immune system reacts to repeated viral exposures as well as how prior infections and immunizations affect future responses.

8. International Cooperation and Exchange of Data:

Initiatives for data exchange and international cooperation are crucial for gaining a thorough understanding of influenza. In order to improve our collective power to combat the virus internationally and to enable a prompt reaction to new influenza threats, future research orientations will emphasize the significance of sharing data, resources, and expertise globally.

These new avenues for research have the potential to completely change how we prevent and treat influenza as the field develops. Through cooperative actions and technological progressions, scientists endeavor to formulate approaches that are not only efficacious against extant influenza strains but also adaptable to potential future obstacles that may emerge in the ever-changing field of influenza virology.

CHAPTER SIX

6.1 Notable Influenza Outbreaks:

Influenza is a respiratory virus that has caused multiple major outbreaks in the past and has had a lasting impact on the global economy, public health, and society. Recognizing the effects of these epidemics helps to reduce the likelihood of such ones in the future by offering important insights into the dynamics of influenza viruses. In this section, we examine a few of the most prominent influenza epidemics in history.

1. Spanish Flu (1918-1919):
One of the deadliest influenza epidemics in recorded history is still the 1918 Spanish Flu pandemic. The pandemic, which was brought on by the H1N1 influenza A virus, killed an estimated 50 million people and affected around one-third of the world's population. Young, healthy adults were disproportionately affected by the virus, and the tight quarters of military camps during World War I contributed to its fast spread. The Spanish Flu brought to light the possibility that influenza viruses could wreak extensive destruction and led to improvements in epidemiology and public health response.

2. Asian Flu (1957-1958):
Originating in East Asia, the H2N2 influenza A virus was the cause of the 1957 Asian Flu pandemic. With its rapid global

spread, the virus is thought to have killed one to two million people. This pandemic brought to light how easily influenza viruses may cross international borders and how linked the modern world is. Increased efforts were made in influenza surveillance and vaccine development to combat new strains of the virus as a result of the Asian Flu pandemic.

3. Hong Kong Flu (1968-1969):

The 1968 Hong Kong Flu pandemic was caused by the H3N2 influenza A virus. It was not as bad as the epidemic of 1957, yet it nevertheless claimed 1-4 million lives globally. The Hong Kong flu showed that influenza viruses with the capacity to spread like a pandemic still pose a hazard. The ongoing investigation of the genetic variables affecting the transmissibility and severity of influenza viruses has been aided by this outbreak.

4. H1N1 Pandemic (2009-2010):

H1N1 influenza In 2009, a virus that is often referred to as the swine flu triggered a pandemic. In contrast to seasonal influenza, young adults and pregnant women were disproportionately afflicted by this pandemic. Widespread vaccination programs were sparked by the rapid global transmission, which brought attention to the significance of readiness, monitoring, and international cooperation in addressing new influenza risks.

5. Avian Influenza (H5N1 and H7N9):

Around the world, avian influenza viruses, namely subtypes H5N1 and H7N9, have sometimes but severely caused outbreaks. These viruses usually spread from birds to people, which means there's always a chance of a pandemic. These epidemics highlight the necessity of efficient monitoring, prompt identification, and containment strategies to stop the spread of avian influenza viruses to human populations.

6. Seasonal Influenza Outbreaks: Annual seasonal influenza outbreaks present a recurring public health threat, albeit not as severe as pandemics. These epidemics have the potential to seriously impair healthcare systems and increase morbidity and death, particularly in communities that are already at risk. Seasonal influenza epidemics emphasize the value of immunization drives, antiviral medications, and public health initiatives to lessen the virus's effects.
7. Lessons Learned and Future Preparedness:

Important lessons concerning the erratic nature of these viruses and the value of international collaboration in tracking, combating, and reducing their effects have been imparted by notable influenza epidemics. Research on influenza, the creation of vaccines, and pandemic preparedness are all guided by these lessons. The necessity for ongoing surveillance, investigation, and funding for public health infrastructure to protect populations around the world from influenza outbreaks is highlighted by the advent of novel influenza strains and possible pandemics.

6.2 Success Stories in Containment and Mitigation

Numerous influenza epidemics have presented significant obstacles to public health throughout history, yet containment and mitigation initiatives that have been effective have also emerged as sources of inspiration and role models for future responses. These success stories highlight successful tactics and actions that have reduced the impact on communities and controlled the spread of influenza by drawing lessons from previous mistakes. Several noteworthy triumphs from previous influenza pandemics are listed below:

1. Hong Kong's Response to H1N1 in 2009:
2009 saw a global outbreak of the H1N1 influenza pandemic, commonly referred to as the swine flu. One common example of a successful response to the pandemic is Hong Kong. Adopting a strong stance, the city closed schools, segregated ill people, and gave antiviral drugs to everyone in the community. The prompt measures implemented by the health authorities in Hong Kong resulted in a comparatively low death rate and restricted the pandemic's overall impact on the populace.

2. Japan's Response to the Spanish Flu (1918-1919):
Strict public health precautions were put in place in Japan during the Spanish Flu epidemic to stop the virus from spreading. Schools were shuttered, mask use was promoted, and quarantine regulations were implemented by the government. Japan's public cooperation and quick response lessened the pandemic's effects, lowering the country's death rate in comparison to some other nations.

3. Australia's Success in the 2017 Influenza Season:
Australia experienced a severe influenza season with many cases in 2017. The nation ran a successful public health campaign encouraging people to get vaccinated as early as possible. Along with other preventive efforts, the campaign successfully raised vaccination rates, which helped to lower the number of influenza cases as the season went on. This event made clear how crucial

prompt and focused immunization campaigns are to contain epidemics.

4. South Korea's Response to H5N1 Avian Influenza (2003):

In 2003, there was an H5N1 avian influenza outbreak in South Korea that threatened the health of humans and poultry alike. Strict control measures were put in place throughout the nation, such as the quick deployment of antiviral drugs, increased surveillance, and the culling of affected chickens. South Korea successfully stopped the virus's spread and avoided widespread human infections by acting quickly and cooperatively.

5. Taiwan's Early and Agile Response to COVID-19 (SARS-CoV-2):

Taiwan's response to the COVID-19 pandemic brought on by the SARS-CoV-2 virus is notable, although not being influenza-related. Taiwan adopted early and forceful steps, including as border control, contact tracing, mass testing, and open communication, in response to the SARS outbreak in 2003. By successfully stopping the virus's spread, these measures reduced the danger to the general public's health.

6. Singapore's Handling of the H1N1 Pandemic (2009):

Singapore put a thorough response strategy into action during the 2009 H1N1 pandemic. Temperature screening was instituted at many points of entry, cases were quickly detected and isolated, and public knowledge of preventive measures was raised. A successful containment of the virus was made possible by preemptive actions in conjunction with efficient communication techniques.

7. United States' Response to the 1976 Swine Flu Outbreak:

A possible pandemic of swine flu threatened the United States in 1976. With the goal of immunizing every member of the public, the government initiated a massive vaccination program. Despite the fact that the pandemic never happened, the vaccine campaign's effectiveness demonstrated the value of preventative public health measures and the capacity to organize substantial resources.

8. Global Collaboration during the H5N1 Avian Influenza (2005-2006):

Countries and international organizations worked together to handle the worldwide threat during the H5N1 avian influenza pandemic. Coordinated measures to cull diseased chickens, information sharing, and surveillance all contributed to preventing the virus from spreading further. The worldwide reaction proved how successful international cooperation can be in stopping the spread of infectious illnesses.

These triumphs highlight how successful it may be to contain and mitigate influenza outbreaks using a multimodal strategy that includes early identification, quick reaction, public awareness efforts, and international cooperation. Even if every outbreak has its own set of difficulties, learning from previous experiences helps to continue developing tactics to deal with influenza and other new infectious diseases.

CHAPTER SEVEN

7.1 Personal and Community Preparedness

In order to prevent the virus from spreading, safeguard vulnerable groups, and preserve public health during influenza epidemics, individual and community preparedness is essential. People can help in the joint endeavor to avoid and lessen the effects of influenza by taking preventative actions at the individual and communal levels. These are important things to think about when preparing yourself and your community:

Personal Preparedness:

1. Vaccination: Give yearly influenza vaccination a priority. A vital component of personal preparedness is vaccination, which lowers the chance of infection and the severity of disease in the event that it is contracted.

2. Hygiene Practices: Stress the importance of practicing proper hygiene, which includes frequently washing your hands for at least 20 seconds with soap and water. If you can't find soap, use a hand sanitizer with alcohol in it.

When you cough or sneeze, cover your mouth and nose with a tissue or your elbow as a sign of good respiratory etiquette.

3. Stay Informed: Use trustworthy sources, like news organizations and public health organizations, to stay up to current on influenza activity in your area.

Observe the advice of health officials when it comes to vaccination campaigns and preventative measures.

4. Stockpiling Necessities: In the event that an outbreak forces you to stay indoors, keep a stockpile of necessities including non-perishable food, prescription drugs, and over-the-counter treatments on hand.

5. Health Monitoring: Keep an eye on your well-being and consult a doctor if you feel like you could have the flu. Early diagnosis and treatment can lessen the illness's severity and stop it from spreading to other people.

Community Preparedness:

1. Community Involvement and Education: To increase knowledge about influenza prevention, symptoms, and the value of vaccines, establish community-led educational initiatives.

Inspire a sense of shared accountability for public health by urging neighbors to assist one another in times of epidemic.

2. Emergency Preparedness Plans: Create and distribute emergency plans tailored to your community that include what to do in the event of an influenza pandemic. This covers policies for public areas, businesses, and educational institutions.

3. Public Health Campaigns:

Launch public health programs to encourage immunization, good cleanliness, and further preventive actions. Communicate across a variety of media to appeal to a wide range of people.

4. Community-Based Surveillance: To track and report diseases like the flu, set up community-based surveillance systems. Timely intervention and containment are made possible by early detection.

5. Assistance for Vulnerable Populations: Recognise and assist vulnerable groups, including the elderly, small children, expectant mothers, and people with underlying medical issues. This could involve community outreach and focused immunization campaigns.

6. Collaboration with Local Authorities:
To guarantee a coordinated response, cooperate with neighborhood associations, emergency services, and health authorities in your area. To improve readiness and response activities, this involves exchanging knowledge, assets, and skills.

7. Training and Drills: To acquaint community members with emergency response protocols, hold training sessions and drills. This improves preparedness and guarantees a coordinated reaction in the event of an outbreak.

8. Encouraging Mental Health: Be aware of the possible effects an influenza pandemic may have on mental health. Put into action programs that deal with social isolation, stress, and anxiety, and offer assistance to people who require it.

Technology Integration:

1. Digital Communication Channels: To share instructions, updates, and real-time information, make use of digital communication channels such as social media, websites, and mobile apps.

2. Telehealth Services: By integrating telehealth services, healthcare facilities can be less burdened during an influenza outbreak by receiving remote medical consultations, assistance, and direction.

3. Contact Tracing Apps: Use contact tracing apps to find and alert anyone who might have come into contact with the infection, allowing for prompt and focused intervention..

Personal and community preparedness for influenza outbreaks involves a combination of individual responsibility, community engagement, and collaboration with local health authorities. By fostering a culture of resilience, staying informed, and actively participating in preventive measures, individuals and communities can contribute to a collective defense against influenza and help protect the well-being of all.

7.2 Mental Health Considerations:

It's critical to acknowledge and treat the mental health issues that often accompany physical health issues in the setting of influenza and flu outbreaks. The significance of a comprehensive strategy for public health is shown by the relationship between mental and physical health. In order to promote mental health during influenza and flu outbreaks, keep the following points in mind:

Recognizing the Effects on Mental Health:

1. Fear and Anxiety: Increased anxiety can be caused by worries about one's own and one's loved ones' health, the possibility of getting the flu, and uncertainty about how the sickness will progress.

Prolonged anxiety can cause emotional suffering generally, difficulties concentrating, and disruptions in sleep.

2. Social Isolation:

Social separation and quarantine are examples of public health interventions that might cause isolation by reducing social connections and escalating feelings of loneliness.

Extended periods of seclusion may exacerbate depression symptoms and a feeling of alienation from social support systems.

3. Stigma and Discrimination: People with influenza diagnoses may experience stigma and discrimination because of misunderstandings about the virus or concerns about spreading.

Feelings of shame, social rejection, and a reluctance to seek prompt medical attention can all result from stigmatization.

Mental Health Support Strategies:

Education and Communication:

Clear Information: To cut down on misinformation and ease anxiety, provide fast, accurate, and clear information on the influenza outbreak.
Access to Resources: Disseminate information about hotlines for support, counseling services, and resources for mental health.

Participation in the Community:

Support Networks: Encourage the development of local support networks to unite people and offer forums for experience sharing and emotional assistance.
Community-Based Programmes: Create community-based mental health initiatives, such as online support groups, to cater to the particular needs of locals.

Training in Mental Health First Aid:

Training Programmes: Provide community members with mental health first aid training, enabling them to identify and address indicators of distress in others.
Vulnerable Populations:
Children and Adolescents: School Support: Make sure that schools place a high priority on mental health by providing tools and counseling to help pupils deal with stress and anxiety.
Parental Guidance: Teach parents how to keep lines of communication open and how to assist their children's mental health.

Seniors:

Telecommuting Social Links: Promote telecommuting social links for senior citizens via technology, mitigating the effects of social isolation.
Health Monitoring: Encourage routine health check-ins for senior citizens, addressing issues related to their physical and emotional well-being.

Frontline Workers:

Support Services: Provide frontline workers with access to mental health support services, acknowledging the detrimental effects of ongoing stress, long hours, and exposure to difficult circumstances.
Acknowledgment and gratitude: Express gratitude for frontline staff members' efforts to improve mental health and morale.

Online Resources for Mental Health:

Telehealth Services: Remote Counselling: By providing remote counseling sessions, telehealth services enable people to receive mental health treatment even when they are socially isolated. Digital Tools: Encourage the use of mental health applications that include coping strategies, mindfulness training, and tools for stress and anxiety management.

Addressing Stigma:

Campaigns for Community Awareness: Anti-Stigma Initiatives: Start efforts that highlight empathy, compassion, and the need to de-stigmatize mental health issues in order to overcome the stigma attached to influenza. Cultural Competence: Provide culturally competent mental health support services that take into account the varied cultural origins and beliefs of their clients in order to promote inclusivity.

Being Ready for Potential Emergencies:

Inclusion in Public Health Planning: Mental Health Integration: Acknowledging mental health as a fundamental aspect of total health, incorporate mental health concerns into public health planning for upcoming influenza epidemics.

Resilience Building:

Community-based resilience programs that enable people to manage the strains and uncertainties brought on by infectious disease epidemics should be developed.

Let's sum up by saying that promoting general well-being during influenza outbreaks requires attending to mental health issues. Communities can reduce the psychological effects of influenza and flu by implementing a holistic strategy that leverages digital resources, fosters community engagement, supports vulnerable populations, and facilitates communication. In order to effectively address the problems caused by infectious diseases, mental health must be acknowledged as a crucial aspect of public health.

CHAPTER EIGHT

CONCLUSION

As we get to the end of our exploration in "Influenza and Flu Challenges: Beyond the Sneezes," it's clear that influenza is much more than just the seasonal illness that people typically think it is. This in-depth exploration of the complexities surrounding influenza and flu problems has revealed a story that goes beyond the simple physical symptoms of sniffles and sneezes.

We've studied the historical records of pandemics, realizing the seriousness of incidents such as the Spanish Flu and how they influenced the development of public health policies. The book has illuminated the many aspects of influenza, from innovative technologies to the tenacity shown in controlling outbreaks.

Our investigation went beyond the lab, highlighting the importance of taking mental health into account when influenza outbreaks occur. An important component of holistic healthcare has arisen as the awareness of the psychological cost and the development of ways to support emotional well-being. The significance of collaborative efforts in reducing the obstacles faced by influenza is highlighted by worldwide cooperation, lessons learned from successful containment tales, and preparation on the part of individuals and communities.

With its emphasis on the need for a proactive and multifaceted strategy in navigating the complex landscape of infectious diseases, "Influenza and Flu Challenges: Beyond the Sneezes" acts as a beacon for informed decision-making. The information provided on these pages aims to equip people, communities, and healthcare providers to meet and overcome the various obstacles these viral enemies present as we continue to deal with influenza.

Sustained investigation, inventiveness, and a unified front against influenza are essential in the dynamic field of infectious diseases. We can work together to get past the sneezes and create a healthier, better-prepared future for influenza threats by embracing information, building resilience, and remaining watchful.